MW01611998

Hospice Patient Stories

LESSONS LEARNED
from
HOSPICE PATIENTS
BILL L. LITTLE, PH.D.

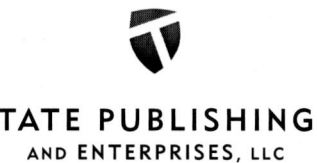

TATE PUBLISHING
AND ENTERPRISES, LLC

Lessons Learned from Hospice Patients
Copyright © 2015 by Bill L. Little, Ph.D. All rights reserved.

No part of this publication may be reproduced, stored in a retrieval system or transmitted in any way by any means, electronic, mechanical, photocopy, recording or otherwise without the prior permission of the author except as provided by USA copyright law.

This book is designed to provide accurate and authoritative information with regard to the subject matter covered. This information is given with the understanding that neither the author nor Tate Publishing, LLC is engaged in rendering legal, professional advice. Since the details of your situation are fact dependent, you should additionally seek the services of a competent professional.

The opinions expressed by the author are not necessarily those of Tate Publishing, LLC.

Published by Tate Publishing & Enterprises, LLC
127 E. Trade Center Terrace | Mustang, Oklahoma 73064 USA
1.888.361.9473 | www.tatepublishing.com

Tate Publishing is committed to excellence in the publishing industry. The company reflects the philosophy established by the founders, based on Psalm 68:11,
"The Lord gave the word and great was the company of those who published it."

Book design copyright © 2015 by Tate Publishing, LLC. All rights reserved.
Cover design by Charito Sim
Interior design by Caypeeline Casas

Published in the United States of America

ISBN: 978-1-68097-319-8
Self-Help / General
15.01.07

LESSONS LEARNED
from
HOSPICE PATIENTS

CONTENTS

What I Learned from Hospice Patients.............................7

What I Learned about Needless Suffering 65

What I Learned about Relating
    to Hospice Patients...79

A Personal Note 91

Afterward or Post Script..97

WHAT I LEARNED FROM HOSPICE PATIENTS

Patient Stories

The stories shared here are true, but several facts are altered to protect the identity of the patients. I want to write this material because of what it means to me. Some of the material that follows will be sad, even tragic. Some will be amusing, even funny. But it all contains lessons I have learned from patients whom I have worked with.

My dad used to tell me everyone is smart about something. Maybe that simply means we can learn from anyone. Certainly there are plenty of lessons we fail to learn, simply because we are not paying attention. I vowed not to miss the lessons patients could teach me. I tell their stories with some of the lessons and affirmations I have learned.

I am still learning from the patients who I am privileged to visit and attempt to help. Patients inspire me and challenge me to be more sensitive to personal needs and to be better prepared to meet their needs as well as mine.

I believe my life has been enriched because of these lessons learned from so many patients and from their families. Perhaps these lessons can help others as well.

These stories are attempts to paint pictures learned from work with hospice patients. Each story begins with a lesson learned from one of these patients. The lesson is followed with a short story about the patients. These are true stories, but the patients will have to remain anonymous. They will, however, never be anonymous to me. I hope that readers will find some encouragement, inspiration, and a little humor from these real people and their experiences.

These are stories taken from moments in the lives of individuals. Note that! Patients are individuals. Each is unique. I have learned that we cannot generalize about people. We often have to report, for the records, that we have seen "a ninety-year-old male with congestive heart failure" or some other disease, as if all ninety-year-olds are the same. They are not.

On a recent visit to see my personal physician for a diagnosis because of fatigue, I was told, "Well, you are a seventy-nine-year-old man. You can't expect to have energy like you did when you were young." Why not? Don't put all of us in the same mold. We are all different.

We need to be aware of the fact that age is not the determining factor. The condition is! When I was twenty-one years old, I suffered a pulled hamstring muscle while running a race in college. I was told it was because I did not warm up appropriately and was given a rehab schedule to repair the problem. When I was in my sixties, I suffered a pulled hamstring muscle while running a race in the Senior Olympics. I was told it was because of my age. I think I may have failed to warm up appropriately, but that was not the diagnosis. It is the condition that is the problem and not the age of the person who has the problem. Of course age is a factor, but it affects each person differently.

I didn't stop playing competitive basketball until after my seventy-fifth birthday. I continue to work out on my elliptical trainer. I work a full-time job and still enjoy traveling with my wife. I know aging affects me but not in the same way it does every other person in my "general" age group. We are all different. No two patients are the same, even if they are the same age and have the same illness. Perhaps in reading these brief stories we can see uniqueness.

I have learned that emotional pain can be worse than physical pain.

One example is the impact of emotional pain, which can be seen in the story of one of the patients in our program. His reactions are different from the reactions of others who have gone through similar experiences, but they provide an insight into some emotional hurts experienced by others.

The patient is an African American and one of fifteen siblings, raised in a foster home (parents were alcoholics). His condition is tragic. He is an MS patient. He says he knows he is dying by inches. His ability to use his body has been reduced to the point that he can hardly use his arms. I have seen him shed a few tears over the awareness of what is happening to him. But I never saw him more saddened or shed more tears than when he shared a memory with me. It was a memory that brought intense emotional pain to him.

When he was an adolescent, he was stopped from picking up his sister from school because of her light complexion. The teacher thought she was white and would not believe she was his sister. He was sent to the principal's office and punished. His foster mother had to come to school to straighten the whole mess out. Tears rolled down his cheeks as he remembered his embarrassment, the unfairness of racism, and that moment of pain in his young life. That experience was symbolic of many other such events for him. His disease mercifully does not create a lot of physical pain, but his memory of the hurt he felt from racism still creates an intense emotional pain.

We should never underestimate the intense pain that comes from emotional distress. As I listened to his memory and watched his reaction, I wondered if prejudice would ever end. At the very least I can let him know that I feel some of his pain and will never let race be a deterrent to our friendship. That gives even more meaning to my work as a chaplain.

This is just one example of emotional pain experienced by patients. A congestive heart failure patient sat in her wheelchair and gazed at the television in her room. She had just told me that it had been months since she had seen her daughter. The daughter lives about thirty minutes from the facility where her mother is receiving care. When the daughter was called, she explained that she had had some health problems but would try to get over to see her mother "sometime" soon.

The emotional pain of loneliness and feeling that people we love have forgotten about us or are just too busy with their own lives to check on us is arguably worse than physical pain. At the very least, it is a pain that should be recognized. Attempts need to be made to help patients alleviate some of that pain. Perhaps our visits can help.

Emotional, spiritual, and psychological pain is real.

I learned that there is tremendous strength in love.

One of the first patients I worked with was a man in his fifties. He had advanced lung cancer and metastasis to other organs. He was so weak he hardly had the strength to speak.

His little grandson was brought in to see him while I was visiting with him. The patient was bedfast and could hardly hold his head up, but he managed to pick the grandson up, lay him across his chest, and play with him. That patient died the next day. Since then I have seen patients exhibit amazing strength in lots of ways, certainly emotionally. I wondered, Where do they get their strength?

I still wonder, but I think I know part of the answer. They get some of it from *love*. When you love a grandson and will not be able to watch him grow up, that love may empower you to pick him up and hold him even for a few minutes.

A common illustration of the power of love is the power demonstrated when an adolescent boy falls in love and no longer has to be told to take care of his appearance and his hygiene. The changes may not last longer than the "love," but they do occur.

Of course, people also get much strength from their *faith*. Believing in God and his grace empowers people to hold emotions together in the face of pain and death.

Some of the strength must come simply from the powerful human spirit with a *desire to live* that is in us all. I continue to marvel at the strength I see in patients. It is not just physical strength, but especially emotional and spiritual strength.

I believe we muster the strength to keep going because we want more time with people we love or we just love life.

11

At any rate, we all have more strength than we realize. I have shared that belief with dozens of patients. I really can relate to their concerns and do not want ever to talk down to them or diminish their pain or fears in any way.

We honestly do all have more strength than we realize and we know that the way through our pain and fear is simply to, figuratively, keep on putting one foot in front of the other. When people add to that natural strength, their faith in God, they discover grace that empowers them even more. But never underestimate the strength that comes from love.

There is strength in love.

I have learned lessons about the value of memories.

Our memories—good, bad, or indifferent—may come back to us during times of serious illness. Sometimes we just need to tell someone about them to enjoy with us or to empathize with us. Sharing memories is often a powerful healing tool. That healing is usually an emotional healing, though not limited to that.

That lesson has been taught through, not one, but many patients. We all like to remember good times in our lives. A visit or a photograph may trigger those memories. Simply asking a question about a patient's past will often give him or her an opportunity to share special times. Memories can be healing.

One patient was an amputee, a victim of a stroke, and congestive heart failure. He was largely confined to bed and often depressed. On a recent visit with him I asked if he had some good memories to keep him company in these difficult days. He did. He shared several of them with me and periodically would smile just remembering. Memory can be bad when focused only on our miseries, but it can lift us up when we focus in on good times.

Another patient was a woman who was often near depression when I saw her. When I asked her what she remembered from her childhood, she became silent for a few minutes then smiled. She said, "I remember going fishing with my father. I was a tomboy and loved to do things with him." She laughed at some memories of fishing trips and said that she even went hunting with her dad.

Her little hands were gnarled into fists from arthritis but her memories were fresh and free. Her memories were her constant companions and when she expressed them her depression was relieved.

When dealing with the grief of those who have lost loved ones, the suggestion that they share memories with their family is often made. It is suggested that they share favorite memories, especially fun and positive ones. What I believed about memories has been confirmed by hospice patients. Good memories make a nice pillow to rest on and can help us gain energy for making new ones.

From hospice patients I learned the value of good memories and would encourage people to share theirs with their families and friends.

There is value in memories.

I learned that though leopards cannot change their spots, people can and often do.

A man can change. He was dying with Parkinson's. He was really afraid to die but insisted that he did not believe in God and had abandoned religion. Nevertheless, he was

13

willing to have chaplain visits because he was assured that as his chaplain, I would not try to change him. We, hospice chaplains, are not to evangelize but to support people where they are.

We visited several times, sometimes in the dining room, sometimes in his room, and sometimes in the hall near the nurses' station. We discussed many things from his life experience, especially his time in military service.

Eventually he began to talk about his fears. The last time I visited him I had been told that he was at a crisis point with his fears. When I got there, he told me, "I am fine. My life has smoothed out. I am ready for prayer and I am ready to die." We shared a prayer time and he expressed gratitude for the time we spent and said, "Hurry back." He has changed!

We are not the same people that we were last year, or even last week or yesterday. We can change, and, thank God, many of us do.

People can change.

I learned again that we just never know what is going to happen to patients.

She was a frail little woman who really enjoyed visits and loved to have the Bible read to her and eagerly anticipated prayer times. She had a sweet and gentle spirit even though she had been abandoned by her family. They had even sold what few possessions she had.

Eventually we were told that she was "actively dying," a term used to indicate that the patient's time was very short. This is a time when we, in hospice, often begin vigils with patients so they will not have to die alone. It is also a time when a chaplain is often called to come and pray a prayer of commitment for the patient as he or she prepares to die. I remember that the prayer time was a very emotional experience for those of us who had been on her care team and for facility caregivers. There was weeping as we said our good-byes. The patient remained nonresponsive. I went away knowing I would soon get the call that she had expired. When I returned the next day, the patient was awake and taking nourishment. It would be weeks before we had another call that she was "actively dying." She rebounded again.

That same experience occurred again in a couple of weeks. As I write this, she is still alive, enjoying visits, loving spiritual input, and "actively living."

A major league pitcher asked once about how his season would transpire said, "I can tell you in two words. 'You never know.'" He has been quoted many times with his two- to three-word response and it really sums up a lot. We never know.

We cannot really ever know when a person is going to die.

I have learned that there is not much significance to what we are called.

The woman has been on the critical list for as long as I have known her, almost two years. She comes and goes as to her condition. Her mind also comes and goes, but she seems to remember her nurse very well and she remembers me, her chaplain. She, however, does not call us by our names. She designated new names for us. I am "Tim."

She remembers. When I miss a visit with her, she will ask her nurse, "Where is Chaplain Tim?" The newly named nurse lets her know that I plan to see her soon.

It really doesn't matter what she calls us. When people have asked me about how they can deal with negative things others call them, I say, "It doesn't really matter. If they call you a tree you will not sprout leaves."

This patient loves me and loves her nurse. It doesn't really matter what she calls us. The old adage that "a rose by any other name smells the same" applies to all. The criticisms and judgments of others really do not matter unless we let them.

Criticisms and judgments of others mean very little.

I have been taught the lesson that we over value material possessions.

A patient who has end-stage renal failure told me recently he has lost all his material possessions because a family member could not afford to keep the locker where he was keeping them. He said there were several thousand dollars' worth of his properties now gone.

I asked him how he was dealing with this loss. He said, "The only thing that really bothers me about it is that I would have liked to give some of it to my friends. The things don't mean that much anyway. They are just things."

I said, "Well, I certainly agree that they do not have the value that we usually give them. The things that really matter are our families, friends, and our faith. I just need to be reminded of that every once in a while. Still I know it is a loss to you."

He nodded. I am sure terminal illness has clarified the values for him but they are the same whether or not we are ill. Things are just things. A new car? It is just a car, a means of transportation. A new house? It is just a place to live. Things run too much of our lives. It shouldn't take an illness to teach us that.

Material things don't matter very much.

A "confused patient" touched me with a lesson about understanding.

I went in to visit this patient who was clearly disoriented. It is tragic to see persons struggling to reconnect with the world outside. I said to this patient, "I'm your chaplain."

The patient responded, "You have chocolate?"

"No, I am your chaplain."

"I want some chocolate."

I was never able to clear the communication.

I went away amused and saddened. It is amusing to hear some mistaken interpretations of words, but I sometimes think they may not be misunderstandings at all but may reveal real, unmet desires. I wished for a box of chocolates and hoped to bring some chocolate to her, but she declined rapidly and died before that opportunity came. We will relate to one another better if we learn to understand from the other's point of view.

Remember, the language of love is always the other person's language. Compassion understands saying Stephen Covey has it right. "Seek first to understand and then to be understood."

A better conversation for the patient would have been, "I am your chaplain." "You have chocolates?" "No. Do you want chocolates?" Looking back on that meeting, I realize that it would have been more important for me to acknowledge her desire than to push for her to understand my role. We need to live in this moment and without judgment. Just relate to one another now! That is a valuable lesson to learn and I learned it from a hospice patient.

So many people are discouraged because they don't believe their opinions and desires matter. They feel "unheard." I want to remember that the next time I interrupt someone who is talking to me. I want to remember that when a patient makes a request. I will at least give a response that will indicate that I have heard what the person is saying.

I wanted to give the patient a chaplain visit but she wanted chocolate. Maybe Forest Gump's mother was right, "Life is like a box of chocolates."

We can learn from everyone.

I learned a lot about relating from an Atheist.

He was suffering from congestive heart failure and was told that he was nearing the end stages of that condition. I called to visit and his wife wanted a visit, but he declined. After a week passed, I called again and she said that he would accept a visit on two conditions. First, I would have to visit him on a Saturday morning (I think he was sure that we worked only five days a week.). I agreed to see him on the following Saturday.

The second condition was that I could not push religion or God on him. I agreed and again knew how important it was for us in hospice to accept people where they are and support them in whatever ways we could.

I met him and enjoyed our conversation very much. We had a lot of things in common, such as shared backgrounds and interests like farming and gardens. He showed me tomatoes that he had raised. He gave me a couple to take home with me. We never talked about God, but at the end of the visit, I said to him, "I respect your beliefs but I want you to know that after I leave here I will be praying for you." He said that would be all right.

Over the next several weeks we visited many times. His health continued to decline but our relationship flourished. We became friends. He taught me clearly that we don't have to agree on faith issues in order to be friends.

When his condition worsened and he was taken to a hospital, I went to the ambulance with him. Before he was taken away, he took my hand and said, "Pray for me all you want to. I need your prayers." I held his hand and prayed a prayer of commitment to God for him. We both wept. He never came any closer than that to expressing faith, but we had established friendship and I know he felt support from me. I never saw him again after that night but I have never forgotten the lesson of unconditional acceptance I learned from him, an atheist, but a fine human being who needed to be supported during the end of his life.

Atheists are people too.

I have learned that even patients who need to be loved also have a lot of love to give.

All of us need love, whether we realize it or not, but most of our patients are very much aware of the fact that they need love. What we sometimes fail to recognize is that they may also want to express their love for others.

I visited a Huntington's patient (Huntington's is an inherited disease in which certain brain cells are destroyed. It frequently results in involuntary and uncontrollable movements of muscles of the body.). She recognizes me now, and when I come into her presence, she says, "Here is my chaplain."

I say, "Yes, I am here to pray for you and your children."

This patient knows that her disease is in her genes and that her children are at risk. She has requested that I pray for her children every time I pray for her. I pray for her and them and she waves her arms toward me for a hug. I am thrilled to have a hug from her and hear her say in her affected speech, "I love you." I love her too. I just wish there was more I could do. The major lesson here may be that as long as we have life, we are not too far gone to give the gift of love to others.

We can all give love.

I have learned to overcome fear through understanding.

A lesson I learned from that same Huntington's patient was not to fear a condition that I do not understand. Her muscles, behaviors, and emotions are not under her control. She flails about and kicks her legs about. At first I was afraid to get close to her. I have discovered that if I get close enough to her, the flailing and kicking won't hit me. I now get close enough to give and receive a hug from her. I am glad I did not miss that. I am not only no longer afraid of this patient's condition, but I look forward to visiting her.

Years ago, I read a book that said, "Feel the fear and do it anyway." Vow to never let fear stop you from doing the things that you either want to do or need to do. Feel the fear and do them anyway.

A lesson for me to remember is that I need not fear things just because I do not understand them. Seek to understand more and we will fear less. When we add love that casts out fear to understanding, we will find ourselves facing life with much more courage.

Fear can be overcome with understanding.

I have learned the value of a relative or friend visiting a patient.

Almost all stories from our patients have more than enough pathos in them. I saw a lonely woman today. Hers is a too-common story like one of the patients mentioned above. She is a veteran of World War II, a Wave for six years. She is in the end stages of congestive heart failure. I asked if there was anything I could do for her. She said, "Call my daughter and tell her that I would like to see her. I miss her."

It has been months since her daughter has visited her. I called but the daughter has simply not felt well enough to visit. I shudder to think of how many similar stories there are. I know people cannot visit as often as they might like, but too often, it is out of sight, out of mind. So many people are simply forgotten. This is another example of emotional pain that exceeds her physical pain.

Remembering this motivates me to keep on visiting, even when I am tired. The people who are confined and sick are tired too. They are certainly tired of being alone. It also motivates me to keep on regularly visiting my mother who is in an assisted living facility. I will not forget to visit her. Visiting the sick is very important.

A simple lesson about eternal destiny.

I was sitting with a patient near the elevators at a treatment facility. We had been visiting for a while and I was preparing to leave. She had really seemed completely disoriented during the time we visited. "I have to leave so I will get the elevator. And the elevator is here now." The doors were opening.

"It is going up and I am going down," I explained.

She said, "Well, we are all going to go up or down someday. It is just a matter of which way you want to go." I believe she was referring to the belief of many that heaven is up and hell is down. Whether or not that is true, her perception seemed to be that it is.

Believing that her reference was about eternal destiny, I smiled at her and said, "I just want to make sure my last trip is up."

She wasn't impressed. She said, "I guess you have to decide." I believe she is right.

Simply up or down, it's a choice.

I have learned that effective communication begins with respect.

This patient is in his forties. His disease (Huntington's) has reduced him to a very thin man who spends most of his days and nights lying on mattresses. The mattresses are lying on the floor surrounded by rubber padding on the walls. The patient usually is lying down, often flailing about with his head covered by a sheet or blanket.

From this man, I have learned that I can only communicate with patients if I respect them and try to relate to them where they are. When I visit him, I kneel on the mattress and then lie down beside him. I tell him I care about him and want to help him. I tell him that all I know to do is pray for him. Sometimes I try to remove the cover from his head but he almost always replaces it. I verbalize prayer and try to express as much caring for him as possible.

It all seems so inadequate but maybe it at least lets him know that someone respects him and wants to relate. I hope he understands. I am sure that he sometimes does understand. He has on at least three occasions responded to my request to pray for him by saying yes. Those were special moments for me. Real communication doesn't require a lot of words and it is grounded in respect.

Respect is essential to communication.

I have learned that there are things worse than dying.

That hard lesson has been brought home to me repeatedly as I work with people in hospice service. I have never been more dramatically touched by this truth than when I met a patient with advanced Alzheimer's.

I walked into his room. He was a dignified looking gentleman, neatly dressed and sitting in a wheelchair. I spoke to him and looked into his eyes. I cannot describe the look but I can tell you that I will never forget it. He looked out at me and began repeating a request, "Help me. Help me. Help me."

I responded with deep desire and said, "I wish I knew how to help you. I will pray for you, but I do not know what else to do." I did pray then and often after that.

"Help me. Help me," he continued to plead. I believe he felt trapped inside himself and wanted help in getting out. I wish I could find ways to help every person who cries out, "Help me. Please help me." If you have an answer, "Please help me."

I am learning that no matter how deeply a person seems lost in his or her mind, they are still there. They are still people, human beings who really want to be helped. If all I can do to help them is sit by them and pray for them, then that is what I will do.

Perhaps there is a greater lesson even than this to be learned. We may be imprisoned by Alzheimer's or dementia, but we can also be imprisoned by preconceived ideas, habits, addictions, greed, lust, tempers, and ignorance. People are working to find cures for the former prisons, but we already know the cure for most of our personal prisons. Patients have helped me to break free from some of my own petty prisons.

This is a valuable lesson, but I still see his condition and believe that if he could not be cured but was destined to live in that prison, it was probably worse than death.

Some things may be worse than dying.

You can't judge a book by its cover.

He was a new patient. He had renal failure and was in end stage. I was told that it would be a difficult visit. He had been in prison two times. His body was covered with prison tattoos, one of which was a swastika.

He was a frail-looking fellow but greeted me with a smile. I introduced myself to him as a chaplain. He did not react. I studied the tattoos and waited for a negative response but none came.

I asked him about his religious background. He gave me the name of his church and his pastor and then told me that he had recently spoken there. During his last prison term, he had become a Christian and did a couple of courses in Bible study.

He was delightful and enjoyed spiritual input and especially prayer. I looked forward to my visits with him. True, his body was covered on the outside with all kinds of tattoos, but his heart was soft with spiritual sensitivity. You cannot tell what is in a person's mind and heart by looking at the outside of that person.

Never judge a book by its cover.

I have learned there are a lot of conditions that imprison people.

I just mentioned some of these prisons in the story above. Perhaps it bears repeating. We can be imprisoned by our attitudes, by our prejudices, by our jealousies, by our greed, by our lust, by our impatience, by our resentments, by our anger, and by our ignorance.

The sad thing about most of these things is that we can find our way out of these prisons if we are willing to make the effort. People who are imprisoned by disease can rarely find their way out.

As I write this, I have been working with three really lovely people who are caught in ALS. One of them is a gracious lady who recently died. She was a gentle soul. I met her six weeks ago when she was sitting at a table in a facility dining room. She asked me to move her glass of water closer to her because she was having trouble moving her hands away from her body. We talked and I spent time praying for her. She appreciated that.

Six weeks later, she was lying in her bed unable to use her hands at all. She barely whispered, "I am ready to go." I have heard that statement many times over the last two years and admit that I often agree with the sentiment. Families are sometimes comforted with the knowledge that their loved one is "better off" dead than to have continued living in such a condition.

No matter how true that may be, we are all reluctant to give up those we love, and the pain of loss is still there. I remind families that though the one they love may be "better off," they will still continue to grieve the loss and that is all right.

A lot of things imprison us.

What I learn about a patient's family and background can help me help them. That has taught me that it is good for me to find out as much as I can about patients.

I recently met a man who was just diagnosed with ALS. He sat in a wheelchair in his living room. Speech was slow. Hand and leg movement was a strain. I asked if it would be all right to pray for him. He said yes. I prayed for God's love to surround him and abide with him no matter what happened. He wept. So did I.

It doesn't take long to love gentle people, and he was one of them. When we discussed his background, he told me that his profession was as a "gemologist." I smiled at

him and said, "You are surely one of God's precious gems."
He smiled.

I was uplifted by that smile. Without some new discovery, his condition will worsen soon. Death may come to him as a friend, but he will remain as a precious gem in the memories of his wife, family, and friends.

It helps to get to know backgrounds, hometowns, children, friends, and issues that have been faced. Was there separation due to time away in military service? Even educational background is helpful when building relationships with patients.

Get to really know people.

**I have learned that people can continue to be
productive even with really difficult conditions.**

I visited once with a seventy-two-year-old man who was dying of esophageal cancer. He is still composing jazz music and he has a perky spirit. It embarrasses me that I get depressed when facing nothing more than legal problems and other trivia. Where is my faith and strength? I really need to reach down deep inside and begin to live as if God is still in control. This patient has the courage to face death…surely I can face difficult times in life.

The point is that he continues life. We can certainly continue living as long as there is life and we can encourage people who are critically ill to continue living. Some even find it helpful to set goals.

It can be a helpful exercise for patients to get specific and write some short-term goals and a few longer term ones. We may ask a patient, "What do you want to accomplish in the next month, next three months, and the next year?" We suggest they think about the goals. Describe them to friends and family members. These dreams or goals may give additional strength and certainly comfort to the patient.

If nothing else, such a mindset reduces the daily stress that accumulates during long times of illness. There is nothing wrong with remaining productive.

Keep on being productive.

That patient also taught me that I can be grateful for a lot more than I realize.

This patient said he has learned to get the most from each day. He is thankful for sunlight shining through the windows of his apartment and for a mail slot in his door where mail is delivered. He said, "I don't even have to go outside to get the mail."

Though he does not believe in God, he tells me he doesn't feel life is unfair to him. He smiles and says, "I have already lived my three score and ten." He is grateful for the time he has had and for the "small" things in his life.

Knowing him has taught me that while I so often breeze by the blessings in my life each day, he is enjoying the smallest gifts. I am learning to be more grateful for even the least of blessings. I have faith in God, but I have learned lessons in gratitude and courage from a man who does not believe in God.

That lesson has reminded me to greet each day with reverence, respect, and thanksgiving. I walk across the threshold of each new day with renewed appreciation for the experiences it holds. That seems to raise the level of my energy and enthusiasm. A patient taught me to remember all of that.

Be grateful.

I have learned again that love is a powerful force.

Funny things happen during visits to sick people. I relate the following story with the notation that what happened was funny but the person in the story is not in a funny place in life. She is a precious lady and I appreciate her. I asked if she believed in God. She said yes. I later asked for permission to pray for her and she granted that. I prayed for her.

After the prayer, she said, "That was a beautiful prayer. I loved that prayer. I love God. I love you, I love you, I love you." She looked up at me with desperate eyes and said, "Do you have a wife?" I could not help but smile. I said, "Yes, and she is a nice lady like you."

If I meet her when we both have our minds about us in the next world, we will have a laugh together about that. I am learning to love my patients, all of them. I love that lady. Finding love in her really inspires me to love others.

Love is a power that bonds us together.

I have learned that connections are inspiring, powerful, and sometimes almost unbelievable.

"Old buddy, old pal." I will never forget the experience with a patient who always greeted me with "Hello, old buddy, old pal." He slipped into a coma two days before he died but would open his eyes periodically.

He had not spoken to anyone for more than two days. I stood by his bedside and told his family about how he had greeted me every time I visited. I repeated the phrase. Suddenly he raised his hand toward me, gently rubbed my cheek, then took my hand and spoke clearly, "Hello, old buddy, old pal." We connected through a greeting. I prayed for him and it was the last time I heard him speak. I believe he spoke once more to his daughter from out of the state when she came into the room. Shortly after that he died.

Patients remember and understand a lot more that we may think. We need to exercise care speaking with them. When we find ways to connect, we have discovered a magic power in relationships. Connecting with them, where they are, is probably more meaningful to us than even to them. When human beings connect with each other, life is enriched and we connect with words, a touch, or even a greeting. "Old buddy, old pal."

Connections are inspiring.

I have learned that real caring is communicated when we speak the same language.

I have a strong conviction that we are better equipped to help people if we can speak their languages. Obviously I cannot learn a great deal of a lot of languages but a little bit of some can help. I have learned a little bit of German, a little bit of Spanish, and am working on learning some French. One language that I have not used much is "sign language."

I did learn enough to do a wedding ceremony for a deaf man but never pursued it beyond that. I now have a patient who is deaf and unable to speak. I went back to the books and learned enough to introduce myself to her, to tell her I was her chaplain, and that I came to pray for her.

After my clumsy attempts at signing, she smiled knowingly and bowed her head for prayer. We had connected! I prayed for her, touching her arm. I stopped touching her at the end of my prayer. She raised her head, smiled, and we waved good-bye to each other. I have never felt much more joy at a visit than I did after this one. I set about learning more for the next visit. I have now learned the "Lord's Prayer" in sign language. I hope I can pray that with her on my next visit.

Learn to speak "their" language.

I have learned that there is power in eye contact.

We all have experienced the discomfort of talking with someone who constantly looks away from us. We doubt that they are really listening to us. That same thing is true of many patients. My experience of that fact came after several visits with an Alzheimer's patient. She had not responded to any interventions made for two months.

It finally occurred to me that I seldom really looked into her eyes. I moved my chair directly in front of her, and literally gazed into her eye. "You do have nice eyes." No response. "I know that you hear me, I can see it in your eyes." She smiled. "You do hear me, don't you?" Emphatically, she said yes. We both smiled and visited. I closed the visit by asking if it would be all right for me to pray for her. She said it would be all right. It was a satisfying visit. It is important to treat people as people and respect them enough to look at them.

She helped me. Since that visit I have been much more conscious of maintaining eye contact with everyone I meet. Maintain eye contact.

I have learned that there is often tremendous power even in our most feeble prayers.

One of the Huntington's patients mentioned above is the young man who flails about on mattresses placed on the floor of his room. He cannot control the motions.

On a recent visit, I lay down beside him on the mattress and began to pray for him. He became perfectly still until the prayer was finished then began flailing. I don't know the dynamics of that, but I will always remember that he was lying still for prayer. There is so much we don't understand.

Years ago I was taught that God will do as a result of our weakest prayers what he otherwise cannot do. I believe that God is empowered by our prayers to achieve his will. They encourage me to continue praying even in my weakest moments.

There is power in prayer.

The child taught me about helping others find their way.

I visited a patient in a poverty-stricken and rather dangerous area. Many of the streets were not even marked and few numbers were on houses. When I went inside and spent time with the family, I apologized for being later than I had promised. I explained that I had been lost.

The little boy, five or six years old, listened intently, and then left the room. He returned with a piece of paper and a crayon. He made several lines and circles on the paper. When I prepared to leave, he said, "Here is a map I made for you so you won't get lost when you leave."

I have tried to keep it but misplaced it somehow. The memory will not be misplaced as long as I live. He is, to me, a precious child. I hope to see him again now that months have passed and see if he remembers drawing the map. I wish we were all as concerned about seeing that we helped others find their way.

Help others find their way.

I have learned that simple things, even trivia, can connect us.

One of the most difficult losses in my time as a chaplain came with a patient who loved football trivia. I used to bring trivia questions to him and he was remarkable with his ability to answer. Once I said, "Do you want the trivia questions first today or the Bible reading?"

He said, "Let's do the trivia first."

After praying for him, I started to leave after a visit. He stopped me and said, "Let me pray for you." In his prayer for me, he said, "Lord, I thank you for Bill. He can't know how much it means to me to have him bring the trivia questions to me."

On another occasion, he asked if he could pray for me again. I said, "Of course."

He prayed but had several pauses in his prayer. He explained the pauses, saying, "I was trying to really pray an eloquent prayer."

I said, "Any prayer for a friend is eloquent." He agreed.

He died today. I found out about it a few hours ago. I have tried to contact his primary care person but have not heard back yet. I am deeply saddened by his death. When we care about people, we are interested in their interests, even trivia.

I ask myself, "Am I learning anything from all these experiences?" I hope so. I hope I am learning more about how to help people prepare for death and about preparing for death myself. I will spend more time thinking about this for as long as I am privileged to live.

Not long after I wrote this note, I was rushed to the ER with pains. After a series of events I had a massive heart attack and was without breath or a heartbeat for more than three minutes. I am just trying to understand what I can apply from that experience. CPR, electric shock, and the grace of God have enabled me to live and to deepen my understanding of my patients. I want to redouble my efforts with them.

Even simple things can connect us.

I have learned that the strong desire to live sometimes keeps people alive.

A male patient went home from the hospital with a negative prognosis. He said, "They say they are sending me home to die and I am going on hospice. I will go on hospice but I will make liars out of them all." He is looking good as of today. He is an example of the people who do well in hospice care. He has been upgraded to palliative care. Palliative care is similar to hospice care except that it is usually administered by hospital staff which provide pain relieving treatment. Usually there is no team to meet social and spiritual needs in palliative care, and patients receiving that care can be upgraded for more aggressive treatment at any time.

We don't have to have a dramatic reason to want to live. We can often release life-giving energy just because we love living. Bernie Seigel once told me, "You don't have to have a reason to live, just a desire. When I ask patients why they want to live, I am most optimistic when they respond by saying, 'I just like to live.'"

Months have passed and the patient is still alive and dong well. He has indeed made liars out of all of those who sent him home to die.

Desire can keep us alive.

I have learned that we can't always help people have their "final" wishes, but we can try.

The patient had vaginal cancer. She was a fifty-year-old woman who, as a result of cancer, had already lost the use of her legs and had been told that she had a "rapidly growing" cancer. When I visited with her she wept asking me to help her arrange to go home to see her family on Thanksgiving. She actually wanted to make the trip on the thirtieth, the Saturday after Thanksgiving. Along with coworkers and contacting her family, we found a possibility, but her doctor recommended we suggest her family come visit her. Nothing was finalized until early Thanksgiving morning. At 3:58 AM on Thanksgiving, the patient died. I hope she died knowing that we were working to help her realize her request.

The fact that she was not able to realize her final wish in no way reduces the significance of the attempts to help her. We fail at times but we must never let that stop us from trying to help the next person reach his or her dream or goal.

We can't meet every wish, but we can try.

I am trying to learn to love God as much as my patients love him.

I envy one patient I saw today. When I asked how she was doing, she said, "I am wonderful. I love God so much, so much. I just love God and I want to do things for him." She expressed her love for God in such real terms that it just has to be authentic. I hope that I can discover that kind of love for God in my life and know it at the time of my death.

I visited her again a month after the first visit. I mentioned to her I really believe that she "loves God." She said, "Oh, I do. I love God. I love prayer. I love you." That was a bonus I had not expected, but it felt good. I told her that I want to love God as she loves him. She said, "God is all we have. He is the most important thing in life."

She is a dementia patient but her expressions of faith are not compromised by her condition. She is real. Her faith and love are real. She expresses wonderful joy from her heart. I love visiting with her. She is teaching me about love, faith, and joy. I hope I can be a source of encouragement and strength to her as her condition declines.

We can all learn to love more.

The lesson of encouragement has been reaffirmed for me.

Patients have unique ways of encouraging and inspiring those of us who visit them. I told one patient, "I'll be back like a bad penny." She said, "On, no. You have such a wonderful smile that you could never be a bad penny." I feel better just having been told that I am not a "bad penny." I want to be more encouraging because it just feels so good to be encouraged.

Another patient I saw today said, "You really love your work and you really love people."

I said, "Yes, I do."

She said, "I know because it shows in your face. You have God's love in you and it shows."

I hope she is right, but she sure lifted my spirits on a rainy day. Dying people often give more to the still living than we can ever give to them.

No one ever died from an over dose of encouragement.

We need to learn not be judge things we don't understand.

A social worker told me about a little Spanish American boy who had been adopted by a very nice family, one of whom had become a hospice patient. The boy was causing commotion in his first-grade class because he talked so much to other students. The parents were called for a conference. The child was asked if he was talking a lot in class. He said yes. They asked him why he was talking so much and he said, "The teacher only speaks English but a lot of the class only speaks Spanish, so I interpret for them."

We all should talk that much!

Don't judge what you don't understand.

I have learned that there may be "dumb" questions.

I saw a patient today who had not been communicating with me. I said to her, "Do you believe in God?"

She looked at me with wide eyes and decided to communicate, "That's a stupid question!" I guess she believes in God!

This patient also reminded me that it is difficult to deal with spiritual issues when there are physical needs not being met. I came into her room ready for scripture and prayer. I said, "Would you like for me to read a scripture passage today?"

She said, "I am cold." She was seated in a Broda chair with a sheet covering her.

I went into the hall and spoke with an LPN who was on duty and asked if there were some covers available for the patient. She pointed me to a stack of thin blankets. I picked up one and went back into the patient's room. I covered her with the blanket and we talked for a few minutes while she was getting warm. Then she was ready for scripture and prayer.

We have to be sensitive to the physical needs of patients when we want to share spiritual input with them. The patient could not be very receptive to a spiritual message while she was shivering in her chair.

There are some dumb questions.

I have learned that people do not fit our molds.

I never know what to expect from patients. This is just one more evidence of the uniqueness of the human patients we serve. One woman, who has been a very difficult visit for me, seldom communicates at all and when she does it is a gruff yes or no.

Dreading the visit, I cautiously went into her room today and as I entered, she pleasantly said, "Good morning." I said good morning to her and then told her that I had come to visit and have prayer with her. She said that would be wonderful.

We visited and then I prayed for her. She said, "Thank you. That was wonderful." I left realizing again that "We never know!" It is a good thing that our job description does not include judging people.

People do not fit in our molds.

**I have learned that love recognizes that
not even our deaths are just about us.**

One patient who I visit wanted me to spend all my time helping his wife deal with his inevitable and imminent death. He knew he was dying and wanted to be sure she is going to be all right through the process. His message to me was to take care of her, nodding toward his wife.

Love is expressed in many ways and powerfully so. Focus on self can stop the flow of love. Love reaches out to help others.

It is estimated that less than 40 percent of dying people have planned for the end of life and the care of their loved ones. This patient taught me a valuable lesson about caring for the people we love. We all need to plan to take care of them!

Taking care of "them" means preparing for death, making plans for the things we want done, writing out our requests, and giving information that they may need at the time of death. Saying I love you means a lot more than using those words. It means acting in caring ways to the people we love.

Even in death we can think of others.

I have learned that a patient's frustration and fear is not necessarily about us.

Patients are not always pleased to see me. Some are not pleased to see anyone. One patient told me to "get away." I moved away from her and asked if that was far enough. She just kept on yelling, "Get away from me." I realized that I did not have to be close to her bedside to pray for her so I prayed from a distance.

Another patient simply told me not to bother her. When I told the duty nurse about it, she said, "You are lucky she didn't take a swing at you."

I had seen these patients before without negative consequences but they, along with a half dozen or so others, don't want to be bothered and they can become belligerent and openly hostile. Patients have a right to reject visits and to express their feelings.

When I was a young boy my grandfather struck my dog because the dog growled at him. On another occasion one of our mules kicked him. He did nothing to the mule. I asked him why he hit my dog for growling and did nothing to the mule that kicked him. He said, "That dog had no business growling at me. The mule kicked me when I walked behind her. It is a mule's nature to kick if you walk behind her. She was just being a mule and I had no business walking close behind her."

I thought about that in relation to patients that I see. They are facing critical, usually fatal diseases. They are away from family and friends when they are in a treatment or care facility. They are lonely, afraid, often hurting, and discouraged. Is it any wonder that they at times lash out? It may just be the nature of people in such conditions. Those of us who are trying to help them must not take such things personally. It is probably just an outcome of their difficult situations. We need to just go back and try again.

It is not all about us. Sometimes it is about the mule!

I have learned that patients remain human beings until they die.

I have at times become too focused on patients as suffering only from their illnesses. They are suffering from other human issues as well. Remembering that will help me to listen and watch reactions more closely.

A seriously ill heart patient was struggling with end-of-life issues. I talked with him about those issues. He seemed to be able to accept what little help I could give him, but he still seemed to be disturbed. I began to rehash the points I had tried to make about facing death. He listened but seemed less interested than at first.

It finally occurred to me that he was bothered by something else. "What are you thinking about?" I asked.

He said, "My wife was in a serious auto accident this week. I think she is all right, but I still haven't seen her since the accident." He was also concerned about his children. He didn't know if his wife had help with them or not. The point is that even though he is suffering from a life-ending illness, he still had other issues like anyone else. He still has concerns about things at home, taxes, bills, children, and his wife, among other things.

We all need to learn not to dehumanize patients, no matter what their diagnoses. We are not dealing with diseases. We are dealing with people. Some of the people we see suffer from Alzheimer's, others suffer from cancer, others have heart problems, some have Huntington's, and there are many other maladies, but all of them still have to deal with all human issues. While we focus on our areas of responsibility, we must remain open to the broader picture and be ready to help or get help for those other areas.

People do not cease to be human just because they are ill.

I have learned that patients can be helped when they are permitted to support others.

There was a patient who has taught me that they can be seen as supportive as well as needing support. People often want to give something encouraging to those who are trying to encourage them. I spent time praying for this woman and started to leave. She said, "Wait a minute, let me pray for you." I waited and she prayed for me, then smiled a satisfied good-bye.

Spiritual support is often a two-way street. We all certainly need support, but sometimes we forget that the source of support may be right in the person we are attempting to help. This was not the last time a patient asked if he or she could pray for me. I have learned that some of the deepest spiritual moments occur when we permit others to help us or "minister" to us.

Permit others to help us.

I am learning that age is not the thing that matters most.

I see patients who are old in years. One of the patients in my care is 103 years old. She is sound in mind and still able to feed herself. I see another patient who is forty years old and unable to feed herself and is often confused about reality.

Illness is not a respecter of age. We have patients in hospice who range in age from early twenties to those a hundred or more.

I challenged my doctor recently when I went in for an examination because my energy was low. He said, "You can't expect too much at this point in your life."

I said, "Please diagnose me as a person and not as an old man." True, I am old by most standards, but I hope I have good health for several years to come. Be that as it may, I, and everyone else, should be treated for their illnesses and examined without limitations of age.

I try to remember that age is not the main factor when I am visiting patients. The patient may be younger than me and still be very ill, or they may be much older and in reasonably good health at the moment. It is not about age. It is about the condition.

Age is not the only issue.

I am learning to listen more closely.

The woman was a patient suffering from serious heart failure and was developing dementia. I started visiting her about six months ago. She impressed me with her faith from the first time I saw her. I sat by her bed in a chair that I would occupy many times over the next several months. I held her frail hand and found that she had a lot of strength. Her eyes sparkled as she said, "I love God." She repeated it at least five times and then looked into my eyes, saying, "I love God, and I love you." I believe she loved everybody, but it was a wonderful sounding statement.

She was to say those words often in our conversations. We talked about her years as a Sunday school teacher and how much she loved the Bible, but she always closed with her "one note." "I love God." A few days ago, I made my last visit with her in this world. She was very weak and I don't hear very well, but I believe she whispered to me, "I love God." I am glad I listened to her.

Listen to what people are saying.

I have learned that people like to share their knowledge.

There is no question that our patients teach us many things. They teach us about courage, courage to face the worst news we can imagine. They teach us about faith. They maintain their faith no matter what happens. Sometimes they enjoy just plain "teaching."

I have visited with an Armenian couple. He was critically ill and she was his primary caretaker. For some reason, I became interested in their background and she asked me if I would like to learn some "Armenian" language. I was interested. Since that time she has had about three new phrases printed out for me at each visit. I repeat them to her husband and he helps me with my pronunciation. The three of us have developed a friendship, beyond my chaplain visits. I treasure my time with these "teachers."

The value of that learning time was seen in visits when he was not being responsive. I would sit or kneel close to him and speak a greeting in Armenian, "Paree lous." He immediately brightened up, and we shared good times together. We generally closed our times together by saying the Lord's Prayer together. I wished I had time to learn it in Armenian but his life ended before we even started on that. Nevertheless I am glad that I was able to be taught by this gracious man.

People love to share their knowledge.

I have learned that strength is more than muscles.

I was called to see a critically ill patient in a hospital. I was told she was very near death and might be actively dying. When I first saw her, there was nothing in her appearance that would alter that diagnosis. She was frail, very weak, and depressed. Her husband stood by the bedside teary-eyed. They were both prepared for the worst. I introduced myself and talked with them for a few minutes and then asked if I might pray for the patient. They were eager to have prayer. We talked for a while longer and I left, expecting to hear at any minute that she had expired.

The next afternoon she was released from the hospital and went home. This changed nothing as far as her prognosis was concerned. The cancer had already metastasized. The second day she was home I visited her and found her to be feeling better, certainly emotionally.

For whatever reason, she began to improve, though still critically ill. She said she was going to trust God and go on. She did.

There was no miracle cure but she did get stronger. A couple of weeks later I went to see her and she was getting ready to go to a beauty shop to have her hair "fixed." I believe it was mostly just to get out of the house, but it was remarkable anyway.

It is now more than five months since I first saw her "dying" in the hospital. I know she has suffered, and I know the disease is still ravishing her body, but she remains unbelievably strong. She never fails to greet me when I visit and always wants me to pray for her. Even in dying, which she no doubt will sometime soon, she exhibits courage and strength beyond belief. What is the point of all this for me? Having watched her live and fight the odds with persistent faith has given me a sense of strength that is available to me when my time comes. In other words, watching this tough lady has given me hope for toughness in my times of crises.

Less than twenty-four hours after I wrote about this "tough lady," she died peacefully in her home. She died, but her legacy will live on through those of us she inspired by her courage and faith.

Strength is not all physical.

We can learn from mentally challenged patients.

There are at least three major characteristics of seriously ill patients. I have learned this while working with mentally ill and PTSD patients. I have learned things that have helped me to communicate with all patients and all others in my life. Think about these three things.

**The major emotion of most
(especially PTSD) patients is fear.**

That is an emotion that we all can understand. We may be afraid of dying, of failing, of being rejected, of leaving no legacy, of being misunderstood, of losing our minds and forgetting our families, or a hundred other things. We all know what fear is but it is intensified in some situations. PTSD patients live with the fear that they will relive the horrible trauma that was the onset of their condition. They sometimes fear going to sleep for fear that they will have nightmares. They have reactions that they simply cannot understand because of the terrible traumas they have faced.

The major goal for these people is safety.

They want to feel safe and secure. Life experiences have robbed them of that sense of security. They are seeking it, but we who try to help them need to recognize that they will have a great deal of difficulty trusting us. We must exercise patience, respect, understanding, and integrity when we are visiting with them. They value safety. We need to remember to respect their needs and their space. Most of them have been pushed too much and the last thing they need from those of us who are trying to help them is more invasion of their space and privacy. I don't want to enter in unless they say it is all right. That is their right.

They try to achieve their goal of safety and security by distancing themselves from people and memories.

They may withdraw in silence. They may physically withdraw from us. They may use anger to keep us from getting close to them. They simply want to feel the comfort of personal safety and security. We are wise to remember that when a patient turns his or her back on us, refuses to speak to us, or lashes out at us, they are probably just trying to protect themselves. When we visit with them we need to remember that none of this is about us. It is about them and their needs.

What can we do? We can treat them with respect, reverence, understanding, and gentle support. Express love to them if it is genuine love. Avoid confrontation and always be honest with all patients. This is what I am learning, and I am just scratching the surface.

What else can we do? We can familiarize ourselves with all the resources available to us. Here are some of them: validation therapy, peer mentoring programs for veterans suffering from PTSD, language interpreters (including sign language).

Here is an example of creative defense:

The patient was a man in his mid-seventies. He was in the Korean War. I asked his wife if she thought he might be suffering from PTSD. She said no. He was not in any battlefield situations. I wondered.

The patient was nervous when any new person came into his area or room. He was ambulatory when I first met him and when a new person came in, he would fidget for a while and then get up and leave the room. The problem became more pronounced with the passing of time.

One day I went in to see him and he started telling me that "he" was in the next room. The patient wanted me to go talk to "him." There was no one in the next room but it soon became apparent that he simply wanted me out of his area. He wants to protect himself by maintaining distance between himself and any "intruder."

The symptoms were becoming more and more pronounced. In situations like that, those of us who are trying to help are wise to move out of the patient's space until, or unless, he or she is comfortable with us. That may not happen but we certainly cannot force the issue.

Perhaps all of us are seeking safety from our fears in one way or another. Perhaps all of us have a tendency to avoid or distance ourselves from the things that threaten us. Maybe we could all be a little more gentle and understanding of one another. I learned this from PTSD patients.

We can learn even from mentally impaired people.

**I have learned that there are times
when we just can't reach them.**

Another patient who was definitely suffering from PTSD protected himself by not allowing anyone other than his nurse or wife to come into his room. I have learned that I can talk to him if I call and speak to him on the phone. That must feel safe to him.

He was a fine man. He was more concerned about the future care of his family than he was about his own. From all I learned about him, he had a history of really caring about others. He was simply afraid. He went off our service before I ever had a chance to relate personally to him. I hope the chance comes again, but often it does not.

In the brief times I visited his home, I learned how important it is to give assurance to critically ill people that we will seek to support their loved ones when they are gone.

I am glad we have a bereavement program that follows our families long after the death of the patient.

We cannot help everyone.

I am learning that patients surprise us.

I am ashamed to say that there are times I dread visiting some patients. I earlier shared my experience with one such patient and I had that dread this week when I entered a facility to visit a patient with advanced Alzheimer's. She had never responded to me in my first few visits. Today was to be different.

When I told her that I was there to talk to her about her faith in God and to pray for her, she shook her head and began to cry. I touched her shoulder and said, "I'm sorry. I don't mean to hurt you at all. I just want to pray for you." She nodded her head.

I spent a few minutes praying for her and when I finished, she reached up with her right hand, pulled my head toward her, and kissed me on the forehead. I felt a little weepy and humbled. I now saw her in a different light and look forward to my next visit with her.

There is something to love in everyone. Be patient and be sensitive. Most people want to be cared for and welcome support, even people in our own families.

Sometimes people surprise us.

I continue to learn to watch for messages people send.

A woman suffering from dementia rarely spoke to anyone around her. She seemed to be losing touch with reality and less and less able to communicate. I have no idea what touched her mind during one of our visits. I know that I was drawn to her with real warmth and concern.

Humor is always an option in visits and most people like to smile or laugh. She was certainly no exception. This patient seemed to be looking for a reason to laugh.

After a time of prayer with her, I asked, "What are you doing?"

She said, "I am minding my own business."

I said, "I like that. Do you know what I am doing?" She said no and I said, "I am minding my own business."

She laughed and said, "Right on!"

We had a normal conversation for about ten minutes. There was laughter and lots of smiles during that time. That experience has been repeated several times since. I have no idea what it is about the time we talk but her daughter, her primary caretaker, remains amazed at her responses.

I said to this woman, "I believe you know a lot more than you want people to know." She smiled at me and nodded mischievously. We might be surprised at how much people who seem demented really know. If we can make contact with them, we may learn a lot.

Listen for meaning.

I am learning to accept "their" reality.

I have been visiting a heart and dementia patient for at least six months. She has gradually withdrawn more and more away from reality but still is very open to spiritual input and seems to understand it clearly. Today, when I saw her, she was lying in bed with a stuffed animal, a dog, covered over and lying on her chest.

51

We had a very nice and connected conversation. Then before leaving, I asked if I could pray for her. She said, "Yes, but I want you to remember to pray for my dog too."

I was fine with that so I prayed for the woman and her pet. After leaving I felt remorse that I had not been more sensitive. I thought maybe she was connecting that stuffed animal to a real pet she had and lost. I will try to find out next time I visit with her.

See from their point of view.

I continue to learn to laugh with patients.

I visited with a really fun lady who has a reputation for complaining a lot. I am sure it is a deserved reputation, but I really enjoy visiting with her and she has always been delightful to me. On a recent visit I decided to sneak in her negative reputation. She had told me that she seemed to have a "bad" attitude.

I told her about a scripture passage that I thought we could benefit from reading. "It is verse 22 of Galatians chapter 5 and it says that when we have the spirit of Jesus in us we will be kind, gracious, gentle, loving—"

She interrupted me and added, "And crabby." She seems to have her own translation! We laughed together at her remark. Maybe a lot of people make their own translations and are just not as honest as she is.

Laugh with everyone.

I have learned that some patients are really helped by music.

Many of us have music stored in our iPhones. We can play that music for patients if they express an interest in it. Sometimes it is remarkable to see the impact of music on patients. At a recent visit with a woman who was dejected and critically ill, it was apparent that she was losing a desire to even talk about her faith or condition. I asked her if she liked music and she nodded.

I started playing "Amazing Grace." Gradually, she began to open her eyes and her lips began mouthing the words. Before the hymn was over, she was singing the words aloud with the music. I asked if she would like to hear another hymn and she was more animated now. She said she would.

I played "Blessed Assurance," and she sang every word of three verses of the hymn and smiled the whole time. Her energy was up and we were able to spend some quality time talking about her faith. I prayed for her and left, grateful that we had connected with the music.

Since that time, I have shared hymns with several other patients, always with their permission. Some do not want to hear it but many are uplifted by hearing hymns they have sung for many years. When we are trying to relate to patients and help them, our motto is "Whatever it takes!" Share the music.

I have learned to listen to patient's insight.

I always enjoyed visiting this one patient with end-stage heart disease. She was beginning to develop symptoms of Alzheimer's. She was having some "time confusion" but most of the time seemed connected to reality. I was talking to her about how much God cares for her. She said she believed that. I said, "Jesus even said that God watches over the sparrows."

She asked, "He said that?" I said yes. She then said, "He sure was clever."

I guess you could say that Jesus was clever. I just had never thought of it in that way before. I went to comfort her and she wound up giving me insight and a fresh thought about Jesus.

Accept new insight.

I am learning to watch reactions to what I say to patients.

It was the second time I visited this particular patient. I shared a passage of scripture with her, played a couple of her favorite hymns from the music on my phone, and then prayed for her. At the end of the prayer, I said, "God, I commit this lady to your keeping, now and forever."

I started to leave when I noticed a pained expression on her face. I asked, "Is something wrong?"

She looked at me with sad eyes and asked, "Are you going to take my life?"

I said, "No. I just want to be supportive to you."

She said, "I'm glad."

I was puzzled by her reaction until I thought about the last phrase in my prayer. I am sure that she thought I was committing her to God, right then. It was almost like a prayer for the sick or the last rites to her.

I am learning to pay attention to reactions. People don't always hear what I intend and I know that in communications intention doesn't mean anything. Results mean everything. What I intended as a blessing and a comfort resulted in causing serious concern or fear in her. That can happen in any communication. It is not what we intend but what results that counts.

Not intention but results count.

Patients may know more than we do.

A patient who seemed to be suffering from dementia said to me, "I am going home and I know when."

I said, "I don't know when."

She said, "I didn't say that you knew when. I said that *I* know when." She enjoyed that. So did I, but still I wasn't sure what she meant.

When patients say they are going home, we sometimes assume that they mean they are going to die and go home to God. That is not always the case. Sometimes they mean that they want to go home to be with their families before they die. Most patients would prefer to die at home. Maybe this patient knew she was going to be taken "home" before she died.

I quote from the Unity Hospice admission booklet. "When surveyed, nine out of ten Americans indicated they would prefer to be cared for in the familiarity and comfort of their residence. The patients' residence may be a private home, group home or a nursing facility. Hospice care helps people fulfill this wish."

At any rate, the patient said she knew when she was going home. She was satisfied in that knowledge. I am glad she is.

We may not know what they know.

Until death do us part!

A couple was admitted to a nursing home facility together. He was experiencing some dementia and at times he really lost touch with reality around him. His wife became ill and had to be taken to a hospital. She had been in the hospital a little over a week when the administrator of the facility received a call from her. She had a personal request. She wanted him to ask her husband to stop telling family and visitors that she had died.

People run into some strange experiences because reality is often distorted. Those situations are humorous but they are also deeply sad. They remind us just how fragile our minds are and how easily we lose touch. We all can lose touch in a flash. We really are wise to express our love and appreciation to one another while we still have our minds clear. We are wise to make our wishes known concerning end-of-life issues.

The wife returned to the facility and he is thankful she is alive.

Death is absence.

Be careful what you offer.

I *enjoyed* visiting a patient who was not sure if he can ever believe in God. I enjoyed him because he was open and honest. After a recent visit, as I prepared to leave, I said to the patient and his wife, "If you need me for anything, please call."

He knew his condition was critical but he maintained a sense of humor. He smiled and said, "I may call you to come and blow out my candle."

From what I have seen and experienced with patients, I conclude that there are many people who amazingly maintain a sense of humor for as long as they live. People who have had a sense of humor seem to keep it.

My father, one of the funniest men I have ever known, had a stroke. It was a massive stroke from which he never recovered. He was in the emergency room of a local hospital. His face was drooping from the stroke and the ER doctor wanted to check the severity of the stroke. He said to my dad, "Mr. Little, can you smile for me?"

My dad raised his eyebrows and said from a twisted mouth, "I could if you could tell me something funny." He never lost his sense of humor. I am still surprised at the keen sense of humor that is in a lot of hospice patients.

We need not lose our sense of humor.

I have learned to focus on my prayers

The patient was a ninety-year-old with stage three Alzheimer's. At times it seems she cannot connect with the reality of the moment, but there are times! This past week was one of those "times." She had chattered on and on about unrelated topics. I stopped her and said to her, "I am going to pray for you now."

She said, "You are?" I said yes. She said, "Well, make it a good one."

She smiled and I said, "I'll do my best."

I thought at that moment how often we verbalize prayer without thinking about it. We may even be able to recite a familiar prayer without giving thought. Because of this patient's request, every time I pray, I want to make it a good one.

Pray good prayers.

I have learned how to grow old.

The patient was a ninety-two-year-old woman with dementia. She only communicated in disoriented phrases and words. That was true most of the time. She was fun for me to visit. We seemed to connect and were able to laugh a lot. On a recent visit, she was lying comfortably in bed. I knelt beside the bed for our visit.

After a few minutes of visiting, I prayed for her and started to rise from my kneeling position. I said, "I am having trouble getting up. I must be getting old."

She smiled and said, "You should go slow on that getting old."

I think that is true but I haven't figured out how to do that. She laughed at her humor. So did I.

Grow old slowly.

I have learned that being ill does not stop some patients from enjoying banter.

This patient was an eighty-five-year-old diabetic with congestive heart failure. She had a reputation for being crabby. My experience with her had been the opposite of that. She enjoyed bantering with me about all kinds of things.

One week when I visited her, I sat down on the side of the bed and said, "I hope I can get up from here. I am getting so old I don't always find that easy."

She said, "You are not old. Look at me. I am 337 years old."

I said, "How in the world did you get to be over three hundred years old?"

Her eyes sparkled. "It wasn't easy!"

I smiled with her and said, "I guess you have learned a lot in three hundred years."

She retorted, "I have learned not to tell all that I have learned." We both laughed.

Sickness need not destroy sense of humor.

I have learned that faith really does make a difference.

One woman was a very pleasant person in her mid-eighties. I say "pleasant" because she always greets those of us who work with her with a smile. This woman was confined to bed and had been for more than a year now. During that time she had lost close family members and two very close friends. Still, there was that smile and pleasant greeting.

When asked how she is able to keep her spirit up, she says, "I have faith in God. I know he is with me."

She was declining in strength but not in spirit. I know she was feeling bad this past week when I stopped in to see her. She opened her eyes, lifted her head from the pillow, smiled, and said, "Oh, hello, Pastor Bill."

She was tired in body but her spirit never wavered. The only explanation I can find for her strength is her clear faith in God. It is possible for us to all have that kind of faith, but it must begin now, not when we are too sick to continue. There is tremendous power in faith.

Faith makes a difference.

I learned never to stop dreaming.

When I first met the man, he was a little caustic and very independent. I didn't know if I would like him or not. As it turned out, he became one of my favorite people to visit. Once one got beyond his tough exterior, he was a warm-hearted man who had a lot of unfulfilled dreams.

One of his most compelling visions was to become someone who helped children adjust to the challenges of school. He just wanted to work with children. He was in hospice care and knew that meant he might have a short time to live, but he never focused on the short time but on the goals he had if or when he got well enough.

After months of visiting with him, I began to catch a little of his spirit. I decided I would continue to dream dreams until I die. I was already in my seventies but my goals and dreams became young. I hope I can convey some of that visionary spirit to those who read these words. Never give up on your dreams and never let your dreams die before you do. We are taught that "without vision, people perish." I believe that is true to the point that real life may cease, not because we physically die but because we discontinue our dreams.

The dreams of some patients are simple and practical (at least in their minds). The most common dream is "to go home." When asked if there is anything I can do to help them, patients frequently answer with, "Get me out of here so I can go home." When they are ambulatory you may find them at an exit door trying to push it open or simply sitting or standing near an exit. This is one more indication of how the research is accurate. Most people would simply rather die at home.

Never stop dreaming.

I learned that patients have rights.

The man with the dream, above, is the same man I visited to get acquainted. I went to his room in a facility and asked about a visit with him. He said, "Not today. I don't have it in my schedule. If you want to make an appointment, I have time next Thursday at 1:30 PM."

I told him that would be fine but my first reaction was negative. I felt a little "put off" by him. On reflection, I realized he had every right to say no to an unannounced visit. I was infringing on his privacy. He had a right to expect that I would honor his schedule. I did. He really made me aware of my insensitivity and rudeness. I seldom have entered a patient's room since then without first knocking on the door (even if it is open) and asking if it is all right to visit. Patients have a right to expect common courtesy.

The fact is, patients have rights that are mandated by law. Some of these rights include:

- the right for respect of property and person;
- the right to voice grievances regarding treatment and care;
- the right to be informed about alternative care and payment resources;
- the right to participate in their own care plan;

- the right to be informed when care plan is to be changed; and
- the right to confidentiality.

Patients have rights.

I have learned the real value of service to others.

The nun had served the church for half a century. She was a gentle woman with an easy smile. She was critically ill when I met her but that is not what bothered her. I started to talk with her about end-of-life issues. She said, "I am ready to go."

Still she seemed depressed, even tearful. Before I could ask her about the tears, she said, "What really bothers me is that I can no longer serve." It was not death that bothered her but the fact that her days of service to the church were numbered. She grieved that she would no longer be able to meet the needs of poverty stricken and sick people.

She truly exemplified the spirit of Christ who said, "The son of man came not to be served but to serve." When we catch that vision we learn that it is service to others that gives the greatest value to life.

Real value is in serving others.

So what's the point?

The point of sharing these examples is to reaffirm that most behaviors make sense when we understand the reason for them and remember that seldom do they have anything to do with us. It is said repeatedly in hospice, "It is all about the patient and not about us."

For me, the theme of all these stories is that patients are still people, unpredictable, unique, and real. They still dream dreams, still feel pain, can still share humor, and have a right to live fully until they die.

Patients have a right to be treated with courtesy and respect.

WHAT I LEARNED ABOUT
NEEDLESS SUFFERING

When I first began my work as a chaplain, I thought it was like an addition to a program designed to alleviate physical suffering. That is still the primary component of what we do in hospice but I have learned that my job is a major part of our work as is the work of each of our team members. I am to focus on spiritual and emotional needs. I have come to understand what Publilius Syrus meant in 42 BC when he wrote, "The pain of the mind is worse than the pain of the body." My job is to help relieve the spiritual and emotional pain of our patients.

I don't know if the word "worse" is appropriate, but the pain of the mind and emotions is as real as physical suffering. One lesson learned from working with patients is that there are times when the mental suffering and spiritual suffering seem to rise above, even the worst physical suffering.

The good news is that much of the pain and suffering that frequently accompanies dying can be relieved through palliative care or hospice care. Add to this the fact that we now know from recent research that most people prefer to die at home, or at least without exotic tubes and needles attached to them. Most people prefer to die with comfort and not being kept alive in pain and suffering. Still, many people are entered into hospice or palliative care much too late to reap the benefits of such programs. The question must be why. Why don't patients come into hospice care much earlier? Let's examine some of the reasons.

1. One reason may be as simple as families are not aware of the desires of their dying loved ones. About 70 percent of people fail to express their desires for end-of-life care. In addition, many families mistakenly believe they are doing the best for their loved ones, young and old, when they continue to provide aggressive and even exotic treatments to patients who are needlessly suffering in a system that too often ignores palliative and hospice care to the terminally ill. When given a choice, most people choose to die comfortably and in familiar surroundings. Certainly that is preferable to being hooked to breathing tubes, feeding tubes, powerful drugs, and other treatment that often fails to extend life and make the final days more unpleasant.

2. Another very troublesome reason for late referrals is that too few treatment people are motivated to make referrals to palliative care or hospice and too few know the benefits of those referrals. A recent study (released in September of 2014 by the Institute of Medicine) blames the failure to make timely refer-

rals to supportive care on "a fee-for-service medical system in which 'perverse incentives' exist for doctors and hospitals to choose the most aggressive care. Still others default to what is called 'life saving treatment' because they worry about liability."

Former US comptroller general, David Walker, said, "It's not an intentional thing. It's a systemic problem. Discussions concerning this problem should begin as early as with teenagers and continue into senior years. Fear to discuss will continue to lead to needless suffering for the dying.

Even more to the point is an article by Nicholas A Christakis titled "Predicting Patient Survival Before and After Hospice Enrollment." He states, "Despite the apparent advantages of hospice care, several barriers exist in terms of patient referral. Physicians' prognoses play a large role in determining when hospice care should begin. Predicting patient survival is a subjective decision dependent on several factors that may vary before and after hospice-enrollment. Currently, the stay of patients in hospice is very short. This can be attributed to late referral by physicians. Additional research on physician behavior and prognostication could help optimize the use of hospice as a valuable health care resource, thereby improving end of life care for terminally ill patients."

Nicholas Christakis, MD, PhD, MPH, is Assistant Professor of Medicine and Sociology, Departments of Medicine and Sociology, University of Chicago. His article can be found on the internet as can copies of the research on "Dying in America," by the Institute of Medicine.

3. A third reason for late referrals to palliative care or hospice care are a number of misconceptions about such care programs. One of the most fearful and damaging misconceptions is that "hospice is a death sentence." This idea flies in the face of facts as reported in an article from Northwestern University by Emily Nelson.

   Nelson reports in the article titled "Hospice Care Can Increase Life Expectancy" (April 18, 2012). She quotes Chicago hospice nurse, Steve Wren, as saying, "There are studies to the effect that show if you are in hospice care your life expectancy is longer than if you are not in hospice care."

   She also refers to the New England Journal of Medicine, published in 2010. A study published in that journal reports that a study in 2010 on terminally ill lung cancer patients showed that those receiving palliative care had a better quality of life and lived an average of three months longer than those who did not receive palliative care. I found similar results in a research project I did at Barnes Hospital in the 1980s. Raising quality of life, reducing pain, reducing stress, and restoring some normalcy to a patient's life has a positive effect on longevity.

Further evidence comes from Nurse.Com with reports that patients are living longer with hospice care. "New research is providing of what hospice nurses have long suspected. Hospice care not only improves the quality of life for patients with terminal conditions but may lengthen life as well." This is according to research reported in March of 2007 in the *Journal of Pain and Symptom Management (JPSM)*. This study confirmed a previous study comparing hospice and nonhospice patients. That study was reported in September 2004 *JPSM*.

The patients who seemed to benefit most from hospice care were congestive heart failure patients. Still, cardiology is one of the more difficult places for hospice to get referrals because of multiple management interventions. Other disciplines have similar reluctance to refer. When more are made aware of these results it may dramatically change the way aggressive life-sustaining treatments are viewed.

There is no question that patients who come into hospice or palliative care are diagnosed as terminally ill and are not expected to live for more than six months. Many live much shorter times than that, but the truth is if patients come into hospice care early enough, they usually live longer than their counterparts who do not receive such care.

The reasons for this are varied and certainly include such things as reduction in debilitating treatment and reduction in pain. People with clear minds who are comfortable are likely to live longer than they would have otherwise. Being informed about this one misconception is exceedingly important because it can reduce the delay of getting patients into service. The tragedy of delay is that the longer people wait, the less chance they have for being helped. People suffer needlessly because they have not gotten hospice or palliative care early enough.

Another misconception that hinders early enrollment in hospice care is the belief that *the only way you can qualify for hospice is if you are presently or actively dying.* What actually qualifies a person to become a hospice patient? One being diagnosed with a terminal disease for which there is no known cure is criteria for admission to hospice. Usually the life expectancy of such hospice patients is six months or less. That does not mean every patient lives that long or will die in that time frame. Many patients begin to thrive when their pain is reduced. We see patients who live much longer than their prognosis suggests. Many patients fail recertification standards and are removed from hospice care. I know of one woman who was in and out of hospice care for two years. She kept getting better in the program. When she failed to requalify, she said, "I guess I have graduated from hospice again."

I have been working with hospice patients for more than a year now. Several things have become clear to me in that year. I am surprised at how reluctant some people are to place loved ones, friends, or themselves into hospice care. Some are still under the misconception that to be in hospice is a "death sentence." That simply is not true. People are going to die in hospice or not in hospice. The fact is that the commitment of hospice to keep people from suffering and enable them to live out their natural life without pain often enables patients to live longer and certainly to live with a higher quality of life.

Another common misconception is that hospice is a place. A hundred years ago that might have been true, but not now. Hospice is not a place, it is a *service*, and that service can be rendered anywhere people are. People receive hospice care in hospitals, nursing homes, rehab centers, and homes. Some people believe that if they accept hospice care it means they must leave their home, which is simply not true. Where one receives care is a matter of choice. It is a choice. This choice is possible because hospice is not a place but a service.

I believe many doctors are reluctant to recommend patients to hospice because of the misconception that they are failing them by making that recommendation. This is no more true than referring a patient to a specialist is failing. None of us can be all things to all people. In the health care profession, we should all recognize that we are on the same team. We are not being critical of physicians because it is common knowledge that they are committed to doing the best they can for their patients. But when a doctor delays referral of a terminally ill patient to hospice care, they are often doing a disservice to the patient and the patient's family. We urge physicians to refer sooner rather than later with the recognition that the patient may opt to return to care if they are not satisfied with their treatment, or if hospice treatment proves to be inappropriate for him or her.

Perhaps the major misconception by families is that when they refer their loved ones to hospice, it is an indication that they do not love them enough to take care of them. The truth is, most people are just not equipped medically, emotionally, or physically to give family members long-term care. Hospice care is really an adjunct to other care that patients receive.

Patients in hospice are given care to remove their pain and discomfort for as long as they live. That is a loving thing to do for anyone, and it is something that hospice workers are trained to do and do even better than most families. It is also true that in trying to take care of a patient's needs without help, many family members wind up hurting themselves.

I recently talked to a really caring woman who was committed to taking care of her mother who had been actively dying for more than six months. This woman was becoming so stressed that she was unable to sleep. She had to find a way to take a break. She decided to place her mother in hospice care. While the care provided did not meet all her mother's needs, it certainly bridged the gap for this family and the mother did well with the care and the daughter regained her balance for living her life as well. This all happened without the patient leaving the home. The care she received from hospice was a supplement to the care the daughter continued to give but could now rely on regular help by trained professionals.

Another common misconception is that people have no choice as to what hospice care they are to receive. Even if a patient is in a hospital that provides hospice care, the patient and his or her family are free to select a hospice of their choice. This fact should be clearly communicated with all patients who are facing referral to hospice care. It is not always communicated by long-term caregivers or hospital staff, and that is a violation of a patient's rights.

The fact that patients and their families can opt for any hospice program that they want often creates competition for patients that put pressure on marketers and staff to enlist patients in their company's program. I work for a hospice program that insists on maintaining a high level of ethics in seeking patients. We acknowledge that most hospice programs are basically good. We do not seek to gain patients by criticizing other programs or people in those programs. We simply try to provide the best service we can and keep our focus on patients needs.

It is mandatory in most states that hospice patients must be provided with nursing care, social work support, and, if they choose, a chaplain, or spiritual support.

The tragic result of misconceptions is that many patients and families who could greatly benefit from hospice care never receive that care or receive it too late. When patients come into hospice care and are still strong enough to communicate their desires and even able to care for a lot of their own needs, like feeding themselves, those patients often actually improve their health. Patients whose families or physicians wait until the patient is near death before signing them up for hospice care do not fare so well. We have patients who are admitted one day and die the next. In many respects, such families fulfill their own misunderstanding that "hospice" is a death sentence. They simply fail to see that the real problem is that they waited too long to enter hospice care.

One final misconception is that once a person is receiving hospice care, they cannot be treated for disease that is not related to their hospice diagnosis. That simply is not true. A patient qualified for hospice as a heart patient can still receive treatment for other problems not related to the heart diagnosis. You can add to this the fact that if you become dissatisfied with your hospice treatment, you may opt out at any time. A patient may decide to try a different treatment program or none at all. Patients never lose their right to choose.

I have been a hospice chaplain. That means that I provided spiritual support and service to any patient or patient's family who desired that support and service. One can be a member of any denomination or religion or no religion at all and still receive chaplain support if they opt for that. It is also true that no patient is required to receive a chaplain's support, but we are to make it available.

I have long been a proponent of the idea that where the kingdom of God exists, pain and suffering are being alleviated. For me that means pain and suffering are to be alleviated for any one experiencing those issues. That includes all people who qualify for hospice care. You have a right to receive service simply because you need it.

How does hospice care work?

Perhaps it will help some to make decisions to receive help if they have a more clear understanding of hospice care. So what is this care and how does it work? Here is a definition:

Wikipedia defines hospice as "a type and philosophy of care that focuses on the palliation of a terminally ill or seriously ill patient's pain and symptoms, and attending to their emotional and spiritual needs." It is a concept that has been evolving for nearly one thousand years. Dame Cicely Saunders pioneered modern hospice services in the late 1950s. Presently, in the United States, the term is largely defined by the practices of the Medicare system and other health insurance providers as a service for inpatients in facilities or in their homes who have a terminal prognosis medically certified estimating that they have less than six months to live. This does not mean that the patient will die within six months. Many live much longer. That is an important note. Surely the research mentioned earlier clearly substantiates this fact.

The definition given here is accurate but it cannot possibly describe hospice and hospice care. Patients are the real definition and story of hospice. That is why I began this book with stories about patients. The definition gives a good general understanding of hospice but a clearer picture can be given by sharing a specific hospice program and how it functions.

Hospice is a holistic program.

Most hospice programs will be similar and we consciously avoid comparisons because we believe that we are all providing a needed service in the best ways that we can. I share Hospice, as practiced by Unity Hospice, because I am familiar with this program. It is a holistic approach to patient care (Most hospice programs are similar to the one we practice.).

The program is designed in this way: patients who come into the program are assigned a team of treatment people. After the doctor certifies a patient for hospice care, a nurse does a physical assessment on the patient and develops a care plan. The nurse is supported by CNAs (certified nurse's assistants). Along with the nurse, they see that the patient's medications are appropriately administered. They also see that the patient is clean and comfortable.

The nurse and the CNAs are joined by a social worker who does a psychosocial assessment on the patient. From that assessment, a care plan is formulated to help the patient and family with information necessary to meet regulations. They are sensitive to the social needs of the patient.

The third component of the team is a chaplain who does a spiritual assessment beginning within seventy-two hours of the patient's admission. The chaplain does a spiritual assessment and develops a care plan for meeting spiritual needs for the patient and the patient's family.

Our teams meet every two weeks to discuss the condition and progress of the patients and any needs we have discovered. That meeting is led by our patient care coordinator and is attended by a hospice physician. Shared information and professional input helps us do a more effective job of meeting the patient's needs.

Note the order of this plan. First, physical pain and comfort are managed. Then social issues are managed, and finally spiritual issues become part of the patient's care. The total program is vital. To borrow from Abraham Maslow's "Hierarchy of Needs," we cannot deal with social and spiritual issues until the physical needs are being met. It is difficult, if not impossible, to deal with psychosocial issues and spiritual issues when the patient is in pain. These issues do not necessarily line up in order. It is possible they may at times be done simultaneously. There are times when it helps the nurse in doing physical therapy to have the patient settled inside spiritually. At any rate, these interventions go together.

A more crude, but effective metaphor is that when you are up to your buttocks in alligators, it is hard to remember that you goal is to drain the swamp. The pressing issues must be dealt with.

Frank Luabach, an outstanding Christian missionary to India, told me that when he was talking with Gandhi about doing mission work in India, Gandhi said they would not permit missionaries to work with the people of India unless those missionaries were committed to helping people with their daily needs before trying to convert them to some other religion. Hungry people need to be fed before they deal with other issues, and hurting people need to have their pain eased before we can deal with other issues.

Our whole program of service is bracketed on the front by Community Resource Representatives whose responsibility is to educate and promote hospice with a goal of encouraging patients to enter our service sooner rather than later. The closer to certification a patient comes into our services, the more we can help them. If the decision is too late and the patient dies within hours or even a few days, we are not able to give them the support they deserve.

On the other end of our hospice care is a bereavement specialist whose responsibility is to be sure that families are supported after they lose loved ones.

Sprinkled throughout our services is another vital group of service people. They are our volunteers. These dedicated people, led by a volunteer coordinator, provide services that range from visits to lonely patients, to pet therapy and music therapy when these are appropriate. They join other staff members to provide vigils for dying patients and assure that no patient has to die alone.

Unity Hospice also provides medical equipment for patients. Our equipment personnel maintain and deliver essential support equipment like hospital beds, lifts, wheel chairs, and oxygen.

Holding the entire program together is an administrator and the administrative staff that works diligently to keep appropriate and adequate personnel in place to provide caring service for all our patients.

We are a team. It is never about individuals. We, like the fabled musketeers, are all for one and one for all in order to keep patients at the center of our concerns. For us, it is all about the patients.

WHAT I LEARNED ABOUT RELATING TO HOSPICE PATIENTS

What I have learned about relating to hospice patients generalizes to all relationships. After all, as I have repeatedly said, patients are just people like all of us. They are simply seriously ill people. The principles of respect, understanding, and relating easily apply across the board to all relationships.

For the first several weeks after I began working with patients, I was struggling especially with those with Alzheimer's. My background in therapy was primarily with cognitive interventions. These did not seem powerful enough for intervening with disoriented people.

I was really emotionally moved with a quote that I read from Schomburg's paper on communication with people suffering from Dementia. The quote from Seneca follows.

> Who is there in all the world who listens to us? Here
> I am—this is me in my nakedness, with my wounds,
> my secret grief, my despair, my betrayal, my pain
> which I can't express, my terror, my abandonment.
> Oh, listen to me for a day, an hour, a moment, lest I
> expire in my terrible wilderness, my lonely silence.
> Oh God, is there no one to listen?

That is what I believe is a description of Alzheimer's patients and may apply to many others caught in a prison of human loneliness. I wanted very much to listen to them but did not always know how. I was elated to discover "Validation Therapy."

I have never been able to see Alzheimer's and dementia patients without really wanting to connect with them. I employed some of the validation techniques from my counselor training but knew I needed more.

A study of the effects of validation on nursing home staff (Alprin, 1980) found administrators reporting that following services in validation, staff began to view disoriented patients as human beings with intuitive wisdom, and not just mindless bodies. This new insight permitted staff to begin enjoying relationships with patients. This in turn reduced the agitation of patients and resulted in quieter floors and fewer restraints and tranquilizers to control behaviors.

I have loved being able to establish connections with critically ill patients with dementia and Alzheimer's disease. I really have enjoyed my patients and look forward to spending time with them. I hope that was reflected in the "patient stories" in the first section of this book.

This general approach of working with disoriented patients gave me a tool to use which helps me relate to those patients. Note that validation gives some important insight and guidelines for working with patients. It is not a set of ironclad rules but a system that provides helpful guidelines for relating to patients. As you will see, most these guidelines provide a basis for relating to people in any walk of life.

We could use other words to describe this approach to therapy. Affirmation comes to mine. We are looking for ways to affirm patients as human beings. Unconditional acceptance is a phrase that also describes this process. We are looking for ways to accept people without judging them. Validation therapy gives us the tools to achieve all these things.

Validation therapy was developed between 1963 and 1980 by Naomi Feil. It was developed to help people with dementia and Alzheimer's but many of us, as noted above, have found this respectful and common sense approach to help not only our patients but to enhance relationships of all kinds.

Centering

Relating to patients should begin with becoming centered in ourselves. This act of centering precedes our contact with patients. If we enter relationships or attempt to communicate with patients without being settled inside ourselves, we will find it very difficult to become focused outside ourselves. Being settled inside enables us to focus on the others. I find it helpful to pause before visits for prayer for myself and to take a deep breath to be sure I am settled inside.

Relaxation is one good stress reducer and a step toward centering. Take deep breaths and internalize your thinking before approaching any important task. Visiting patients is for me an important task. When I am at peace inside, I can more effectively encourage peace in patients.

We are taught in hospice to focus on patients and their needs. Dealing with our own anxieties before visits is essential for establishing helpful relationships with our patients. We set our own anxieties aside for our time of visiting. Centering can enhance relationships with coworkers, friends, and family, but here we are focusing on care for hospice patients.

Preparation is vital. We want to be prepared to affirm or validate the patient (and, coincidently, to be able to validate all with whom we come in contact).

In a paper on communicating with parishioners with dementia, Roger Shomburg says, "The basic technique of validation is to listen intently to what is being asked or said, to accept the person as they are, to not try to fix them up; and to stop arguing to try to change their mind. To listen in such a way as to avoid confrontation with the individual's reality is the ultimate goal of validation."

When patients come into hospice care, they will be helped immediately if we can validate them as persons, real valued human beings. Medication will relieve physical pain but only acceptance and validation will help patients find peace within to meet the challenges of their situations.

It becomes incumbent on all of us who work with hospice patients to understand techniques that validate and to have a real desire to apply these techniques in our contact with patients.

The Patient's Reality

Once a caregiver is "centered" and relaxed, that caregiver is ready to communicate "understanding" and acceptance to the patient no matter what the patient's physical, emotional, spiritual, or mental condition is. Reality orientation insists upon orientation to present-day reality. Validation respects the reality of the person even when it is not related to the present. Validation is based on the belief that there is logic behind behavior and that logic may not be related to present-day reality.

A man suffering from dementia said he saw a man coming across the street to visit. The man had been deceased for more than forty years. The patient's wife had known the man the patient saw coming across the street. His reality moved him to a time when he wife was still living. His disoriented mind had its own logic. There was reason behind his thoughts. It was his way of dealing with his grief.

Seeing the patient's reality really does help us understand and relate to them.

This process of accepting the reality of the patient may be designated as the second phase (after centering) in validation therapy. Sometimes patients cannot differentiate between present and past reality. To understand their communications or behavior, it seems most helpful to identify their reality.

Patients may be disoriented to the point that they have trouble recognizing or accepting reality. But remember that their reality has logic behind it. The logic may not match our logic, but it is real to them. An example I read is of a disoriented man who, as a child, had been punished and embarrassed for either bed-wetting or wetting his pants. He is now at the physical stage of being unable to control his bladder. Instead of facing the problem, he blames his roommate for spilling water on the floor around him or on him.

This patient's reality enables him to deal with wetting on himself without feeling the brunt of embarrassment and blame. To that man, his reality justified his problem.

In such a circumstance, it is not necessary or even wise to clarify the blame but to begin helping by cleaning up the "water." That can be preceded or followed by saying, "Don't worry about it. We'll be able to clean this up and if it happens again just turn on the call light."

When the nurse or aid does not get upset but is encouraging, the patient feels less apprehensive and is likely to feel validated or accepted. He is not as likely to look for blame when this happens again and success will be achieved with that patient when he comes to the place he can say, "Looks like I did it again." The response is still the same: "It's all right. We'll just get this cleaned up and you can be comfortable again."

Until the patient reaches the point of accepting reality, the validating caregiver accepts the patient where he is and even lets the patient communicate by venting or symbolically dealing with the issue. The patient at least needs someone who will listen with empathy and acceptance. A person is validated by acceptance.

Probably all of our relationships would be enhanced and of higher quality if we accepted one another where we are and listen to one another without judgment and rejection. We all need to be validated with acceptance.

Too often we enter relationships with a goal of fixing the other persons misconceptions and ideas. In short we too often try to turn others into replicas of ourselves. If that is a goal you will not be effective in a healing relationship. Accepting the other person's reality is essential to establishing a healing connection.

Using Nonthreatening Factual Words

This process employs a technique described as "using nonthreatening factual words to build trust and acceptance" (phase three). Instead of arguing with the patient described above, the use of factual statements is helpful. "The floor is wet and you seem to have gotten wet too." If that statement is made without a judgmental tone and followed by empathy, "You must be uncomfortable with being wet so let me help dry you up and I'll clean up the water. Just relax and let me help you."

Give the patient freedom to respond from where he is without being critical of him. That freedom is validating to the patient.

Paraphrase

A fourth phase of validating can be simply learning to rephrase the statements of patients to communicate understanding. The patient is wet and blaming his roommate. The caregiver can respond to the patient's accusations by saying, "So you believe someone spilled water on you." That is reflective communication and lets the patient know that you are listening and understand. He begins to feel validated.

We can get into reflective listening by beginning a response by saying, "It sounds like you are saying." For instance, "It sounds like you are saying that someone spilled water on you. Is that right?" The patient is then free to say, "Yes, someone spilled water on me." It is counterproductive to argue or try to correct the patient's perception. Just accept the perception and begin to build a relationship of understanding without judgmental statements. Be patient with the patient and I know that requires centering in ourselves.

Polarity

A fifth technique is the use of extremes or polarity. "Is this the worst thing that has happened to you this week?" The patient can say it is or can continue to vent his frustration with the situation.

A patient I often visit seems to always complain about the terrible food being served wherever the patient is. Stating extremes produces polarity that enables the patient to complain without being reproached. A sample response of polarity would be, "Is this the worst food you have ever had?" Maybe yes, or maybe a worse meal is remembered, but either way, the patient can feel freedom to express.

Imagine the Opposite

A sixth technique of validation is "imagining the opposite." The conversation can continue with a question like, "Are there times when he doesn't spill water on you?" The patient can respond with acceptance of the fact that there are times when this doesn't happen and once again feels validated.

One patient said, "No one at this place likes me. They all avoid me all the time." Imagining the opposite would be, "Can you think of anyone who likes you." Or you might say, "Can you imagine that there are some people who may like you." Moving away from concrete statements to "possibilities" is often at least helpful in engaging in conversation.

Share Memories

A seventh approach may be the use of implementing memories. "Can you remember times when you woke up dry?" Remembering better times can be done while still accepting the situation of the present. The patient is still not threatened and feels validated.

The patient who believes no one likes him may be asked, "Can you remember a time or place where you were liked by someone?" Such nonthreatening statements can help to establish communications.

Eye Contact

Obviously different situations call for different uses of these techniques and may even call for some other interventions. One that has often been helpful for me is "maintaining eye contact."

When a patient is explaining or complaining, or just venting, looking into his or her eyes lets the person know that you are paying attention and really care about what they are saying. Do so without judging the person. Acceptance is the goal here.

Use the Patient's Terminology

Another intervention that can be helpful is to incorporate the patient's terminology. This is especially helpful in trying to communicate with disoriented patients whose comments make no sense or are completely out of touch with reality.

One patient I have seen is almost always disoriented and dramatically so. She will sit and cry for her mother hours on end. She may remain in that state of confusion, but it also may help to relate to her by saying, "You really miss your mother, don't you?" If she is calling her "mama," use the patient's terminology, "You really miss your mama, don't you?" Our goal is to validate the patient and relate to him or her.

Speak in Clear, Low, Loving Tones

Another technique we try to follow for all our patients is to use a clear, low, loving tone of voice. If the tone is harsh, disoriented people may become angry or withdraw. A low tone is best because many patients have difficulty hearing and low tones are usually more easily heard.

Tone of voice is important in most interactions. Some people respond more to the tone of voice that to circumstances and words. "Why are you speaking to me in that tone of voice?" Or, "Don't speak to me in that tone of voice."

Tone of voice that is soft and clear can make messages much more acceptable when we are trying to help someone deal with incongruent thoughts and actions. "Why are you doing that?" can sound like an accusation or an honest attempt to understand, depending on the tone of voice.

Mirroring

There is also a method that can be used but is in my opinion most helpful for the caregiver. It is mirroring the expressions, tone of voice, and posture of the patient. This may help the patient to feel understood, but it will certainly put us in touch with what the patient is feeling. In other words, it will help us to be more understanding of the patient's state and that will help us connect with our patients.

Connect Behaviors to Needs

Another technique that can be useful is linking behaviors to needs (the need for love, for a sense of being useful, or to express feelings or thoughts are some basic needs to be linked to behaviors). A behavior may seem unusual, out of place, irrational, but it usually is linked to some need. Folding a piece of paper may be a desire to be useful by folding something like a towel or pillowcase.

Identify Lead Senses

A very important relational technique is identifying the patient's lead sense in communication. This is a means of learning the preferred communication language of the patient and speaking that language. The language of love and caring is always the other person's language.

The primary languages are visual, auditory, or kinesthetic. People use words that communicate visual ("I see," "I get the picture," "Show me") preferences. They may use words that communicate auditory senses ("I hear that," "Now listen," "Tell me what you mean"). They may also use kinesthetic words ("I feel," "That doesn't grab me," "I sensed that"). If we respond with their language, we will make a connection with them.

Validating caregivers often use gentle and nonthreatening touch to make a connection with patients. If there is any sign of resistance to the touch, stop it because it is not appropriate for that person.

Use Music

Finally, we also use music when it is appropriate to help patients remember or just to let them enjoy something that is meaningful to them. We may take iPhones with music recordings and ask patients if there is any kind of music they enjoy then play that, or if the patient cannot communicate, we play some music and watch for their reactions.

Any technique we use in working with a hospice patient is for the purpose of validating the patient. Their feelings, actions, thoughts, and experiences are valid for them. We want to communicate respect and caring for patients and try to do that through techniques of validation therapy.

We need to use these methods until they become almost like second nature to us. They become natural and flow easily in our conversations. We need to practice until we know these approaches and are comfortable with them.

I sometimes sum up all these techniques as expressions that enable us to show respect and reverence for the people with whom we are working. We are learning to speak the language of respect, reverence, and love.

An Orientation Suggestion

Hospice workers could benefit by role playing. It could be helpful to include role playing as a part of orientation for new caregivers. We could take turns playing the part of the ill person and the caregiver. This would give us a chance to practice validation therapy and become more comfortable with it.

No matter how good we become at treating patients, we will never be as effective as we could be until we learn more about communication.

A PERSONAL NOTE

I was privileged to work with hospice patients for nearly two years. I have never had a job that was more fulfilling to me. I really fell in love with most of the patients whom I worked with.

I can still feel the gnarled, arthritic hand of an end-stage heart disease patient when she reached out to me and held my hand. While holding my hand, she prayed a prayer giving thanks for my visit and for my caring for her. You can't find much more warmth and love than that.

I can still hear the whisper of the little lady who was dying when she said, "I love God and I love you." I would not take anything for memories like that.

I loved walking into rooms of people who were having a bad day and seeing them smile and greet me. There was nothing shallow or meaningless in the pleasure they showed in their greetings.

There is no more pleasant feeling in the world than standing or kneeling by a patient for a time of prayer and hearing the patient's reaction, "Amen and God bless you." If you ever have a chance to have a similar experience, don't miss it.

I told the stories because I believed the lessons learned and affirmed by those patients could inspire people who are struggling with their lives. But I also recorded them because they will be a reminder to me of the joy I had in working with hospice patients. I thank God for that experience.

I woke up this morning thinking about what I learned from working with hospice staff and patients. I honestly believe my life has been enriched through this experience. For me this has been a God thing. I didn't plan on being a hospice chaplain, but when I became one I thought I wanted to do that for the rest of my life.

That was not to be because of circumstances beyond my control created by past mistakes. Still, even that situation can work for good just as my retirement from my pastoral role did in the past. My critics and judges have placed me in a position that has given me a chance to see the redeeming power of God's grace more clearly. My work as a hospice chaplain took so much time and energy that I would never have been able to finish this book without time off. Patients showed me by example that good can come from bad. This confirmed again what the scriptures teach, that all things can work together for good if we stay committed to God.

Now, what have I learned that really enriches my life and raises the quality of my existence for my remaining time?

I have learned that life is really fragile and uncertain. It will definitely end soon and could end at any time. I have known this intellectually for a long time, but now I know it experientially. I really know it now! I have sat by bedsides of dying people thinking that I would not see them again only to find them recovering the very next day. I have sat by the bedsides of others who seemed to be doing quite well and received a call telling me that they had died that very night and the family needed my support.

This knowledge has led me to write my end-of-life directives. This is something all of us would be wise to do. The people we love and leave behind at death deserve to know what our wishes concerning health care, end-of-life care, funeral, and memorials are. I have seen in hospice care many people fail to do this and their families suffer as a result. I have seen others who have taken care of this task and seen their families benefit from knowing their wishes.

I have learned to value things differently. Most things don't matter very much. I told a story about a patient who lost almost all his material things. He discovered what I am learning. They don't matter that much. What matters and what I am learning to value more every day is being alive with opportunities to do something worthwhile. I value the time with the ones I love and my friends. I value the opportunity to share who I am and what I can do with others. Beneath it all, I value the grace of God and his loving care in my life. I want every day to do what I believe is the guidance of God in my life.

I have learned that the end of life is not a thing to be feared but embraced as a part of the natural order of things. People in our care have taught me this with their attitudes of acceptance and peace at the end of life. I learned it from my own brief encounter with death (for three minutes). When CPR brought me back, I realized that if I had not been brought back it would have been all right. I want to live and be productive for as long as I can but hope I can embrace the end at the right time as a good thing.

I have learned to really care about people. I listen more intently, watch faces and actions more closely, accept more unconditionally, and respect others as people of real value. Seeing everyone as someone of value is something I have believed to be right for a long time and have taught clients to see themselves as having as much value as anyone else but this teaching has become a reality for me, for myself, and others.

Part of seeing the value of others is in seeing it in patients, but it is also in seeing it in coworkers, family, and friends. Every person who is making an effort to help others do what is best in their life is special. I respect and appreciate nurses, administrators, office personnel, CNAs, social workers, equipment people, marketers, and facility staff as vital to making life better for us all (I should add chaplains to the list as well).

The list of valued people goes beyond the work place and the family. It includes people in all professions and walks of life. It includes the people we see every day in places of business, on the highways, in hospitals, in schools, and on and on. People are valuable.

Directives

An advance directive is a written instruction that expresses an individual's wishes regarding health care when he or she is unable to make treatment decisions. The intent of the advance directive is to enhance the individual's control over medical treatment decisions.

These directives include a living will, a durable power of attorney, a health care proxy, and whether or not a patient wants resuscitation when the quality of life is gone.

It seems to be a wise thing for patients who are going into hospice care to make a complete list of advance directives for their care. This would be given to the hospice staff and kept in their medical records file.

One of the questions asked in directives for end-of-life care for me was "If you are diagnosed with and incurable disease with limited time to live and if you would not be able to maintain memory of people you love would you choose conventional treatment to prolong existence through feeding tubes or would you choose hospice care?" I choose hospice care.

As indicated above, I believe it is a loving thing for us to do when we leave instructions about end-of-life care, funeral preferences, and memorial service instructions. There is no need to leave difficult decisions to our families during what will already be a difficult time.

I have had some really great teachers in my years of education but I have never had a better group of teachers than the hospice patients who I was privileged to work with. I went into my work as a hospice chaplain with the idea that this would be something I could do during the last years of my life which would be fulfilling. I loved helping people, and this was a field that was ripe with people who really needed help.

What happened was not really expected. I was able to help a lot of people over a two-year period, but I never helped any of them as much as they helped me. I went into the job to teach others and wound up being taught. I hope that readers will at least catch a portion of the inspiration and lessons I received from my work. There are tremendous lessons to be learned from hospice patients. I wake up every day with thanks to God for another day of life and for the privilege of having worked with so many wonderful people, staff and patients.

AFTERWARD OR POST SCRIPT

Reflecting on the experiences that led to this book and the lessons I have learned from hospice patients reminded me of the work I did for ten years with cancer patients. I was program director for the St. Louis Cancer Support Center and saw more than a thousand patients and their families over a ten year period.

One of the things I did with patients was try to teach them the principles that I had learned doing research with cancer patients at a local research hospital. The lessons learned in that study involved eight interventions to help patients respond more positively to their treatments.

Patients were taught to never lose hope. Hope energizes and helps people maintain strength for responding to treatment. Patients were taught to keep on pursing their goals both short term and long term. Goals have a way of drawing us to them and giving us motivation for living. They were taught to practice positive and healthy thoughts. They were taught to exercise and eat healthy diets. Patients were also taught to envision themselves as healthy and to maintain a strong spiritual life that included forgiving others of wrong doing and maintaining a spirit of faith and love. All of these were valid and helped our patients in their treatment programs.

What struck me as I looked back at my experiences with the hospice patients was that I seldom tried to teach them. I tried to support them, pray for them, encourage them, and then I started learning from them. Strange as it might seem, it had not occurred to me to learn from my cancer patients but it became a major part of my relationship with the hospice patients that I saw.

In retrospect, the overall lesson for me was that we would be wise to learn from one another. We probably spend too much time telling others what we think or what we think we know and not enough time listening and watching for lessons that we can learn. That has changed a lot of my life and I wish that I had been wise enough to begin learning earlier.